super *sex* positions

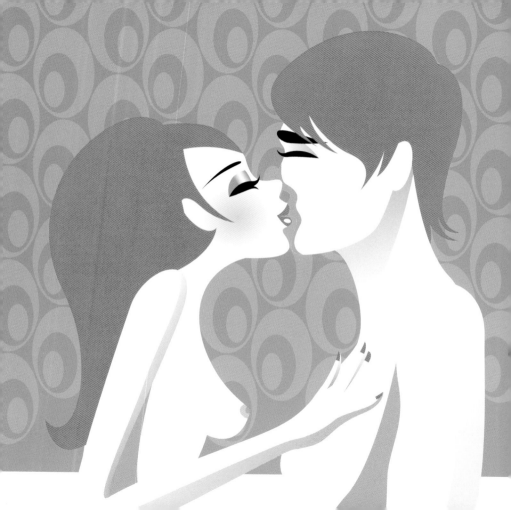

super *sex* positions

paul scott

illustrations by pinglet@pvuk.com

RYLAND
PETERS
& SMALL

LONDON · NEW YORK

Designer **Vicky Barclay**

Senior Editor **Catherine Osborne**

Production Manager **Patricia Harrington**

Publishing Director **Alison Starling**

Illustrations **pinglet@pvuk.com**

First published in the
United States in 2008
by Ryland Peters & Small, Inc.
519 Broadway, 5th Floor
New York, NY 10012
www.rylandpeters.com

10 9 8 7 6 5 4 3 2 1

Text, design, and illustrations
© Ryland Peters & Small 2008
Text by Paul Scott: pages 10–49, 62–63
Text by Sophia Mortensen: pages 52–60

ISBN-10: 1-84597-562-6
ISBN-13: 978-1-84597-562-3

Printed in China

contents

introduction

"Not tonight darling, I've got a headache" are words that we all dread hearing in the bedroom. Recapturing the excitement you both experienced during your first few months as new lovers requires both imagination and stimulation, but this can sometimes be tricky to initiate without a bit of a guiding hand.

When routine creeps between the sheets, it's important to make sure you spice things up by adding a bit of variety to your sex life, and what better way to do this than by introducing a few new moves. If you're a slave to the missionary position, why not let the woman take control by letting her have a bit of fun on top. Try doggy style if you're feeling a bit more energetic and fancy a thrill. For those looking for something a little more daring, there's always the slightly more adventurous sounding Bareback Rider, Scissors, or Vice—moves that will have you in positions you never thought possible! For more advanced couples, choose from a sizzling selection of kama sutra techniques to get your pulses racing. Tips and tricks along the way will soon have you perfecting your performance in the bedroom—from the best positions to stimulate her G-spot to how to press all his pleasure buttons. And don't forget to play safe in the bedroom (see pages 62–63).

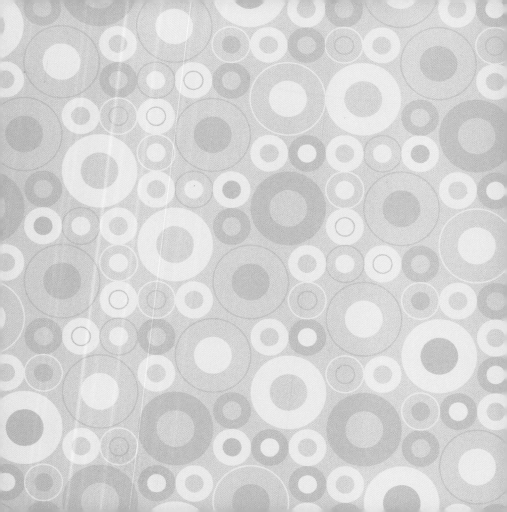

chapter
one

new twists on old moves

missionary position

This is the most common sexual position, of course, and the one most of us think of first. Its reputation for being boring, however, is undeserved. Just because it's the most natural position, that doesn't mean it has to be lazy sex.

She lies on her back with her legs parted; he lies over her, supporting his weight on his elbows and thrusts once he is inside her. It's part of the fun if it takes a guiding hand. Missionary sex offers little for the woman who wants to take the lead, and it's not renowned for offering great clitoral stimulation. However, there are ways of maintaining her clitoral arousal despite the fact that missionary sex offers most of its sensation vaginally.

Placing a pillow or cushion underneath her hips alters the tilt of her pelvis, opening her clitoris to much more friction against his pelvic bone than when she is flat on the bed. If you are both enjoying a slower pace of intimate missionary sex, then an alternative to the man burying himself to the hilt in his partner involves him withdrawing slightly as he continues to thrust, supporting his own weight, and slipping a hand, palm downwards, gently down her stomach until his fingertips find her clitoris.

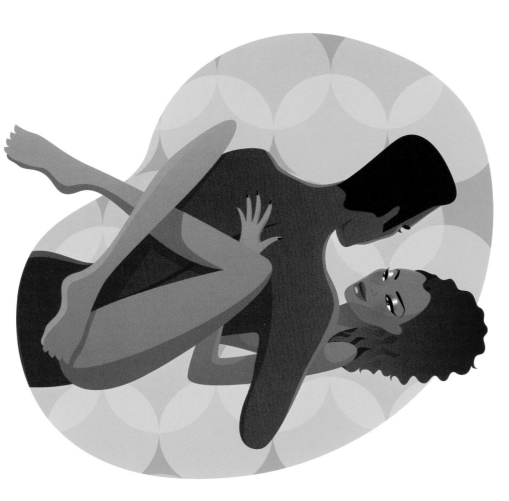

legs inside

This variation on the missionary will spice it up: she lies on her back and spreads her legs so that he can penetrate her. Once he's inside, however, instead of wrapping her legs around the outside of his, she slides them down so that they're straight, running inside his legs, like closed scissors.

This position can lengthen her vagina, making for a new range of penetrative feelings (and accommodating him better if he's extra-well endowed); squeezing her legs together will stimulate her clitoris, and she can squeeze against his penis with her vaginal muscle more strongly than when they're apart.

Using her hands, she can push his buttocks until he is deeper inside her. Otherwise, she has less control than in many positions, which makes this position fun if she enjoys a feeling of helplessness. With her arms by her sides, it's ideal for a bit of light-hearted bondage.

i surrender

From a kneeling position, she leans backwards until she is lying on the bed with her legs folded beneath her. She may raise her arms above her head as he lies on top of her. Her breasts are stretched taught, sensitive to his touch and the skin of his chest, and meanwhile other parts of her body, such as her sides, are more accessible than usual to his touch.

he kneels

She lies back with her buttocks on the edge of the bed, while he kneels on the floor in front of her. The bondage and SM (sadomasochism) possibilities of this position, along with those described previously and below, could include strapping her ankles together using cuffs, which she could then use to draw his head towards her; or else she could toy with his nipples and chest with her feet, while wearing heels.

the "flower press"

She lies back and he kneels on the bed in front of her with his legs parted. She brings her knees right up to her chin, so that her feet are on his chest, or over his shoulders and either side of his head. With his knees on the bed, either side of her buttocks, he is perfectly placed to enter her from above. Particularly deep thrusts are possible in this position, since her pelvis is tilted upwards, allowing for maximum penetration.

She can pull him more deeply into her by clutching his hips, and use her feet—if he likes that—to play with his nipples, chest, and neck, or have her toes sucked. It is easy to reach each other's bodies when making love this way and, although kissing is impossible, there's plenty of space for talking, laughing, and smiling. Her body in particular is more exposed than in the conventional missionary position, especially her breasts and clitoris.

the car hood

As a variation on the position above, she lies back with her legs in the air and her buttocks at the edge of a table, counter, or even the hood of a car, while he stands in front of her. This is great for taking sex outside the bedroom. If he is standing, he is especially free to position himself for maximum stimulation of her G-spot; and to grind and rotate his hips, moving his penis around inside her. This position can't be beaten for fast, opportunistic lovemaking. She is thrillingly open to him. However, she's also prone to being pushed backwards, and may feel vulnerable, so he should take care to hold on to her.

female missionary

He lies back while she climbs on top of him, facing forwards, supporting her weight on her forearms, her legs extended behind her. Moving her whole body up and down will massage his penis. She can press her legs together to increase clitoral stimulation, or fan them outwards, forcing her hips further onto his shaft.

This position won't work at all if there is a big difference in your heights, and while some men enjoy the tease of moving to her pace, others aren't so keen. However, this is one of the only woman-on-top positions where you're intimate enough to kiss and talk throughout. Both of you can enjoy skin-contact all over your bodies, and natural erogenous zones like the breasts are turned-on. His pubic bone will grind against her clit. She is free to stop the action for a second or two, to delay his coming. This is a great position for him to enjoy if he likes restraint during sex. Tie him up, or cuff his arms to the bedposts, and pleasure yourself on top of him!

face-to-face

The simplest way to get into this position is to roll over onto your sides from a conventional missionary position with him on top, maintaining penetration as you go. Otherwise, you can try to achieve it by edging closer, face-to-face and on your sides, with her raising her uppermost leg to allow penetration.

Take care not to squash each other's thighs. This position doesn't allow much thrusting, and may frustrate some couples, although that remains true of side-by-side sex generally, so this is no exception. Although penetration may be shallow, not only does this position allow great intimacy, it requires it, since if either of you let go, you may end up rolling backwards when he slips out of her. Meanwhile, you can kiss, caress, and talk dirty to your hearts' content.

For the adventurous, try holding yourselves together at your stomachs if possible, with a wide belt or straps. Massage oil (and a surface you can clean afterwards) takes this position to new heights of sensation.

spoons

She lies on her side, and he snuggles up behind her. She draws her knees towards her chest, assuming a slightly fetal position, and opens her thighs as he tucks his knees behind her, entering her from the rear. Once he is thrusting inside, she can raise and lower her topmost leg for greater or lesser penetration.

Penetration can feel a little shallow for some couples, especially if their sizes vary greatly. However, it's a great opportunity for him to indulge the sensitive skin of her ears, neck, and shoulders, whether kissing, nuzzling, or using his hands. He can whisper those horny stories or messages of love in her ear, and this position is perfect for intimate, sensuous sex. With her cradled in his arms, this position also suggests those traditional, protective, and protected male and female gender roles. You don't even have to move to float blissfully off to sleep afterwards. Try cuffing or loosely tying your ankles to each other's to add a thrilling element of bondage into an otherwise safe and secure position.

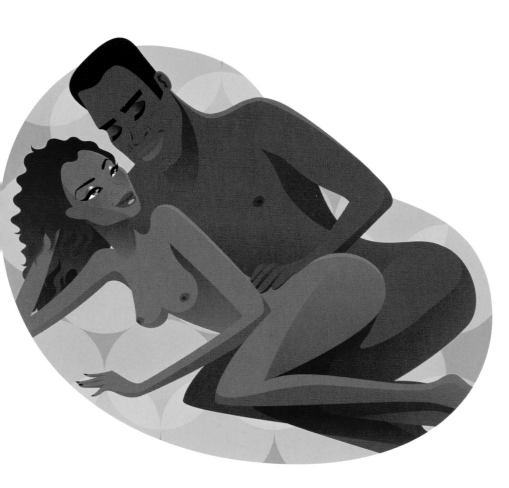

the wraparound

She lies on her back, with her arms and legs open. Rather than lying on top of her, he crouches above her. She wraps her arms and legs around his shoulders and back, pulling herself close around him, and him deeper into her. Pillows or cushions beneath her hips and back may lessen the strain in her arms and legs.

He may feel that his thrusting movement is limited as she clings to him, and he needs strong arms, legs, and back to support her weight. And, as both partners are using their hands for support, loving touch is precluded. However, lots of constant movement is possible with this position. The thrusting, rocking, and inevitable changes of angle ensure that his penis enjoys tip-to-root stimulation, while he is more likely to deliver some stimulating strokes to her G-spot than in conventional missionary sex.

the doggy

She kneels on all fours, either on her hands or elbows, her legs slightly parted. He kneels behind her, his thighs at right angles to his calves, which rest along the bed or floor. He penetrates her vagina from behind, holding onto her hips to push and pull her onto him in time with his thrusting, or to steady her and hold her still so that he can enter as far as the base of his penis.

This is an intense buzz for the man, and it's not uncommon for him to come quickly in this position. Some women find it impersonal, while others, by contrast, relish being taken this way—it depends entirely on the individual. If his penis is larger than normal, she may feel overwhelmed by the depth of penetration possible.

The angle means that his penis is well placed to stroke backwards and forwards against her G-spot, on the front wall of her vagina. You can reach back with one hand and stroke your own clitoris as he thrusts. While he has a great view of his penis pushing and pulling in and out of her vagina, she can move in time with his rhythm as he places his hands gently around her hips, trading off control with him and finding out precisely where the experience is at its most intense.

doggy, standing

She leans forward against a wall, or holds onto something such as a banister or railing. He gets behind her and bends his legs until he's low enough to penetrate her from the rear. Alternatively, she can bend far forwards, holding onto her ankles, or even onto his for support. His hands on her hips and buttocks can also help here.

This is fast, furious, and animalistic. With her legs slightly together, her closed buttocks act to increase the clutching effects of her vagina, making penetration tighter and stimulating her labia and inner thighs. For him, the feeling of her buttocks being closer together is as if her vagina were longer, and penetration deeper.

This is a great position for a short time, and very energetic. It can become difficult to balance, though. It is best to be near a variety of anchored fixtures you can safely grab hold of. Not all couples are ideally suited to this when it comes to their relative heights. It's best if he's fully erect before entering her, and he may or may not enjoy the sensation of having his penis pulled slightly downwards. If she takes to this, she can reach behind her and grab his buttocks, pulling him as far as possible into her. With more movement, he can see his penis sliding in and out of her, while she is free to fantasize.

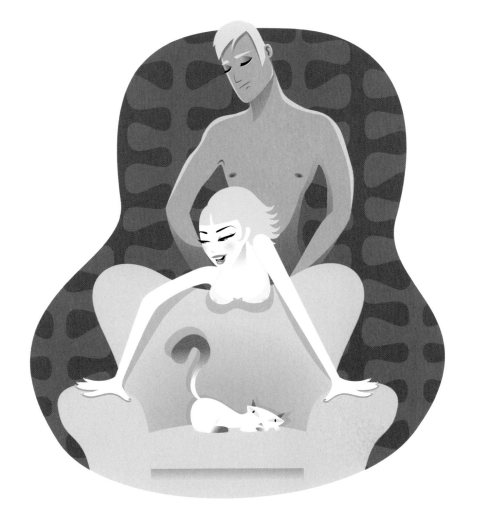

chapter
two

hitching
a ride

ride 'em, cowgirl!

He lies on his back. She straddles him and slides herself down onto his erection. She uses her thighs to move up and down. Unless she has an athlete's thigh muscles, this position can get tiring quickly and can induce cramp. Some women don't enjoy the exposure involved in this position, while others relish the break from being the one underneath, or even being squashed.

Meanwhile, some men prefer to be in control of the pace of the thrusts while others can feel vulnerable that they will slip out and suffer an injury if she rises up too high. Most men, however, relish the sight of their partner's pleasure and her bouncing breasts, which their hands can reach and play with. He can also use his hands to guide the pace to one he prefers, if he wishes. Or, with his hands under her buttocks or on her hips, he can help to push her upwards if her legs tire. This position is great during pregnancy, to avoid squashing her womb. More generally, this is a fun position for exhibitionists, and it's perfect for showing off a new sexy or kinky garment or set of lingerie. He'll want a pillow behind his head or else his neck is bound to get sore from staring up at you.

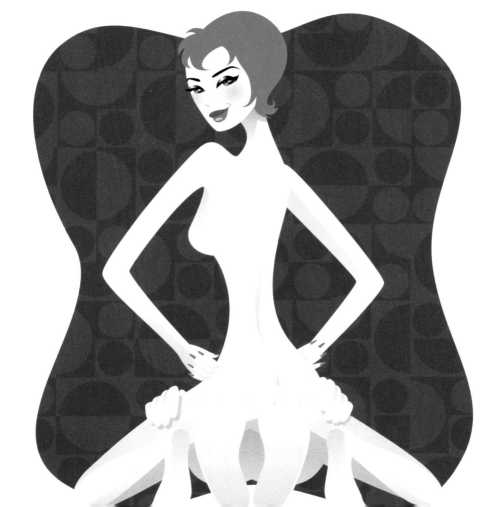

bareback rider

If you're not up for "ride 'em cowgirl" (*see* page 26), then give this position a go, but facing in the opposite direction. He lies back and she squats over him, facing his feet, and slowly lowers herself onto his erect penis. She leans forwards, on her hands, and moves up and down. Or else she can lean back over his chest so that they are lying cheek-to-cheek, almost able to kiss, teasingly.

It can take a while for both partners to get comfortable in this position and, what's more, it offers little clitoral stimulation for her through penetration alone. If she's leaning forwards, he can't reach her clitoris, but she can stimulate it herself. There's little work here for the man; however, if the woman is leaning forwards, he is free to play with her buttocks, anus, and perineum. If she leans back, he can reach her clitoris and breasts. When she's leaning forwards, there's an anonymity to this position in which both partners can let their fantasies run wild. If she's leaning backwards, on the other hand, the position is curiously intimate and novel. Either way, it's the only position that combines the thrill of rear-entry sex with the perfect fit of woman-on-top sex.

"x" hits the spot

He lies back on the bed, supported by pillows, with his legs apart, while she lowers herself onto his penis. Then she very slowly leans back until she's lying backwards at a similar angle to him, with her legs extended, either side of his shoulders. From above, the two of you should look like the letter "X."

Be careful! His penis will be in a new and strange position, its upper surface moving more firmly than usual against her pubic bone. Penetration will not be as deep as usual for him and, since the top of his glans curves away more than its underside, his penis is more likely than usual to pop out, painfully.

That said, you can both enjoy great eye contact, and penetration is very visible this way: you can both see the penis sliding in and out of the vagina—a big turn-on. Penetration feels unusual for both of you, and the sense of not being able to move much can actually be a real tease, rather than the frustration you might expect. You both have plenty of space, if either of you is likely to get claustrophobic, while a mirror on the ceiling will unleash any sleazy-motel fantasies!

scissors

He lies back on the bed or floor and she squats over him, facing his feet. She slowly lowers herself onto his erection. She then leans forward, extends her legs behind her and slowly rocks up and down on his penis. She can't lie still because the angle of her vagina around his penis would bend it too much. And this isn't the position for her if she's not confident about her bottom.

However, her weight bearing down on him creates an incredibly snug fit. She can squeeze his penis with her buttocks during intercourse to make penetration feel even deeper, and can grab onto his legs as he thrusts, to keep her balance. The more she shifts around, the more different parts of the penis and vagina can be stimulated. She can lean onto his thighs if she's worried about being too heavy for him. For a novel pleasure—either for him or for her—he can play with and suck on her toes during lovemaking.

the human chair

He sits on a chair with his legs together. She sits on his lap, facing away from him, and lowers herself backwards onto his penis. He is held down by her weight and so she must do most of the work, rocking and thrusting to maintain arousal.

His penis is at just the right angle to stimulate her G-spot, and both of you can reach her breasts, nipples, tummy, and clitoris. This position is fun, but tiring for her upper legs. By grinding her hips into his lap, burying his penis to the hilt, and moving in a circular motion, she can minimize some of that strain.

Since both of you are looking in the same direction, and she is so exposed, this is a great position if you are watching something that turns you both on, or are facing a full-length mirror. From this position, it couldn't be simpler to move to another, such as doggy-style (*see* page 21), so it makes for a novel way to start making love.

the vice

He sits on the floor with his legs extended in front of him. Gently, she inches into his lap and onto his penis, until she can settle her full weight on him and wrap her legs around his back. The couple sit facing each other, with their legs crossed or wrapped around each other's backs. In this position, you can slowly rock yourselves to orgasm, hugging, massaging, or scratching at each other's backs.

It can be hard to balance, but as long as you don't let go of each other, she's in control of the thrusting. However, the sensation of all her weight bearing down on him will compensate! She'll need to inch a good deal forward against his tummy if she's going to take him inside her to the hilt. Using all her weight can make for massaging penetration. She may enjoy setting the pace and how deep she takes him, while he may enjoy doing less than he's used to. Because of the way her legs are spread, the skin around her clitoris is stretched thinner than usual and is extra-sensitive to the touch. Being so up close and personal, you'll find yourselves kissing and whispering to each other. She can reach between his legs and play with his scrotum, while he can reach her clit. If he's feeling strong, he can cross his ankles underneath her buttocks, which playfully makes for a little more "spring."

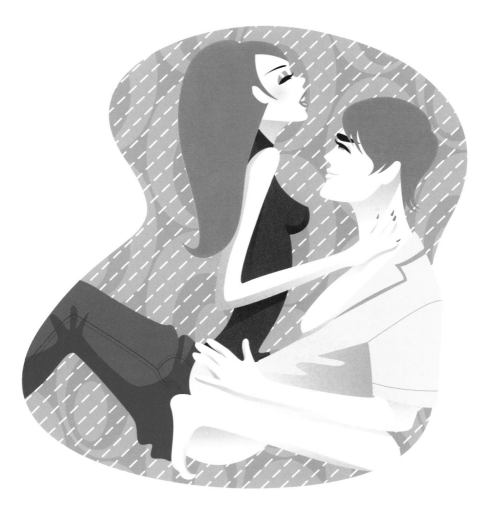

the hinge

He sits in a (well-made!) chair while she straddles him, her knees up, so they're level with and on either side of his chest, and the soles of her feet are flat on the seat, either side of his thighs and buttocks. She holds onto the back of the chair and pushes away with her feet, moving up and down on his penis. His hands are free to explore the whole of her body, from her shoulders and breasts to beneath her buttocks, while this position can be both intimate enough for you to kiss and caress and vigorous enough for you to scream the house down.

She may feel that if she relaxes too far onto him, her body weight will feel heavy on his thighs and put him off. Over a longer time, her thighs may get too tired for her to come. He can help with this and can master the rate of her movements, by placing his hands on her waist or under her buttocks and gently guiding her. Her nipples are in the perfect position for him to nibble and suck as she bounces up and down. As well as being fun and intimate, this is a great position for a quickie—and all the better because it's probably not the one you first think of.

snakes

This is another great position in which you're very likely to come together! The aim is to move at the same pace in the same way: it is based on pressing and rocking techniques rather than the thrusting we're used to. He is on top of her with his knees together against the bed, not dissimilar to the missionary position, but with his pelvis directly above hers.

Instead of thrusting from beneath, his penis straight, his penis is curved, and his hips are riding high. His penis is inside her, but its base is just outside her vagina, and his pubic bone is pressing down on her pubic mound. She wraps her legs around his thighs and rests her ankles on the backs of his legs. Keeping their arms and legs still, they push into each other at precisely the same rate and speed.

This depends on a rolling and rocking motion rather than thrusting in and out, in the way we've all become used to making love. Be patient, however, and this can be a real treat for her as her clitoris presses against him; he will enjoy the teasing delay while being very sensitive to the orgasmic contractions of her vagina. This position delays male orgasm, increasing the likelihood of your coming together.

chapter
three

if you dare

the "Y"

She lies on her side facing him, with one leg in the air and the other flat along the bed. His lower leg slides against her lower leg while her raised leg rests on his shoulder and he penetrates her from the side.

With thighs easily squashed and hip-bones easily bruised, this isn't an ideal position for making love on a hard floor. Balancing can be difficult, and he'll find it more natural to stab jerkily, and more of an effort to establish a steady rhythm. However, it is really visual and playful, and lets you reach towards each other and watch and gaze at each other. He has a great view of his shaft sliding in and out of her vagina, and you both have a visual feast in each other's face and body. He can also reach and play with her inner thighs.

This position can be playful and fun, especially if you both like the idea of messing around with a video camera, and because her legs are so wide apart, she is very open to him. He can really experiment with the strokes that feel best, from gentle, shallow penetration, to deep, powerful thrusts.

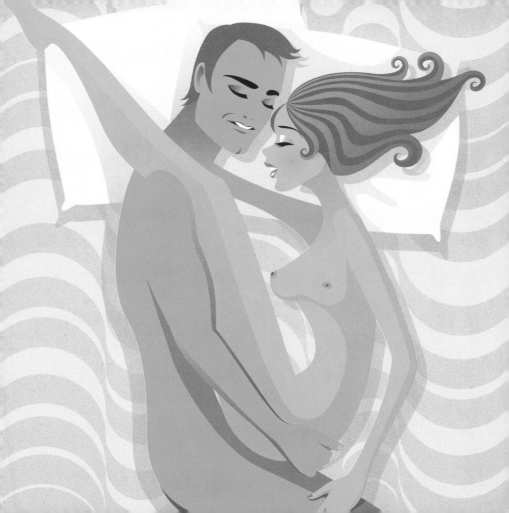

the professional

He sits up on the bed with his legs drawn slightly towards him.
Straddling him, she lowers herself onto his erection, wraps her
arms around his neck to balance, and hooks both of her legs over
his shoulders. A slow, rocking motion is bound to lead you both
to pleasure.

If you find it hard to balance, try this position with him leaning
back against the headboard. She'll need to be supple in order
to keep her legs in place throughout your fun. If you both like
vigorous thrusts, this won't be the one for you; however, it is very
intimate—you're wrapped up in each other, and it's easy to talk and
kiss throughout. It also combines deep penetration with access to
her clitoris, and is gentle, sensual, and slow. He can kiss and stroke
her legs throughout, so this position's great with a pair of sexy
stockings or boots.

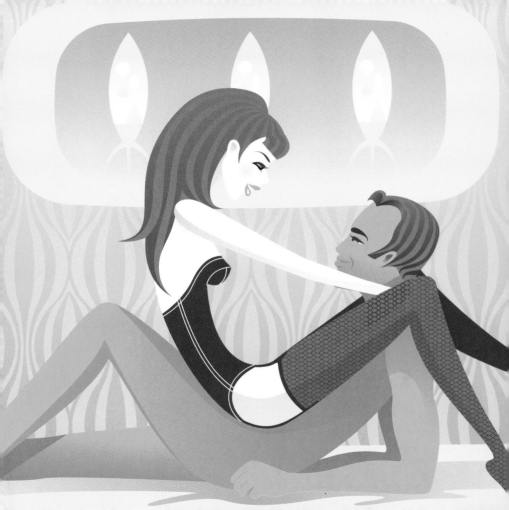

the here and now

This is the position of choice when you just can't wait until you're next near a bedroom! She sits on a surface about the same height as his pelvis. He stands in front of her and unzips his fly or—to avoid a tell-tale "ring of confidence" from her arousal— drops his pants and underpants completely. As he penetrates her, she brings her feet around to the small of his back and wraps her legs around him.

This is great in the kitchen, garage, or after hours at the office, but if there's no available worktop or desk, you can make love up against the wall. This offers less support for both of you, and will require some strength on his part, with his hands beneath her buttocks.

The thrill of a quickie can accelerate the woman's sexual response, and she may come more quickly than usual. Alternatively, her body may not provide lubrication quickly enough to make for easy penetration, no matter how excited she is. In this case you might wish to try some lubrication if convenient, but otherwise, the point is to have fun, so do something else!

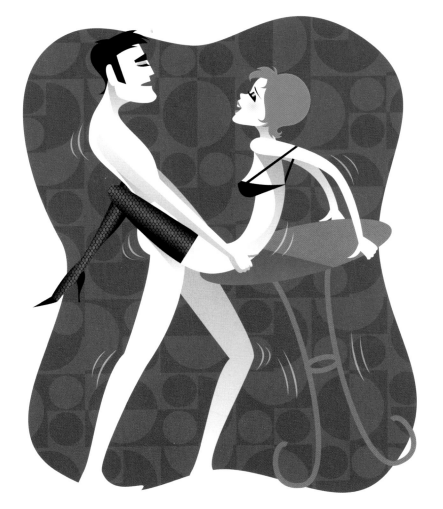

the living bed

He lies on his back and she allows him to enter her, either by crouching onto him, facing his feet, or by lying straight back on top of him, facing upwards, to begin with; in this case his penis may need a helping hand to enter her. She can either rest her legs along his or to each side of his with her soles flat on the bed or floor; or even, for a particular twist, tuck her legs beneath her so that her feet are beneath her buttocks. Her thighs will ache, but, for a short while she'll be able to "bounce" a little, and exercise a little control.

Penetration isn't especially deep but it's very effective: for him, there is extra pressure on the underside of his shaft, while she can experience her own hands together with his as they caress, tease, and pluck at her taut breasts, nipples, tummy, and open labia. She can also bring herself off with her fingers as quickly or as slowly as she likes. He has total access to her breasts and clitoris too. He will find he can thrust for a long time in this position, especially if she's much lighter than him, providing a steady bedrock to the highs and lows of her arousal. Because she is facing away from him, and because the base of his penis is pushing against the back wall of her vagina, he'll feel the deliciously intimate contractions of her anus and perineum as she comes.

standing ovation

He begins by kneeling (he may find this easiest when beginning on one knee), and she lowers herself onto his erection, facing towards him. As she does so, she wraps her legs around his hips and puts her arms around his neck. Cautiously, he rises until he is standing up, carrying her with him and beginning to bump and grind his hips as he does so.

Don't worry if you can't take more than a minute in this position. It's just a fun, spicy twist that you can use to reach a position that offers some support for her buttocks, such as a counter, as he tries to stay inside her all the while. This is a position that appeals to traditional gender roles, with the man taking charge; she will not be able to govern movement much and is dependent on his bouncing her up and down to move on his cock at all. One variation that gives her an element of control is if he stands with his back to a wall, a foot or so away from it. She then has a surface to push against with her feet.

This is a fun position that can make you both feel sexy—if you do sustain it long enough to come, there's enough skin-on-skin contact between you to make this extra-special.

halfway up the stairs

She stands on the stairs, facing away from him and in an upwards direction. Standing behind her, he enters her. He'll find what follows easiest if he places one foot on the stair above his back foot, with the rear leg straighter than the one in front.

Once he is inside her as far as the base of his penis, he circles one arm around her belly and, with the other arm, takes hold of her leg, just below the knee. Carefully, she takes one leg off the stair, gradually allowing him to support her, stretching her vagina around his shaft. If she feels confident enough in his strength, she can raise her other foot too, as far as is comfortable, and reach her arms behind her to touch his hips when she feels he has her whole weight. This will shift her center of gravity backwards and upwards, putting more of her weight on his arm around her tummy and making it easier for him to hold her that way.

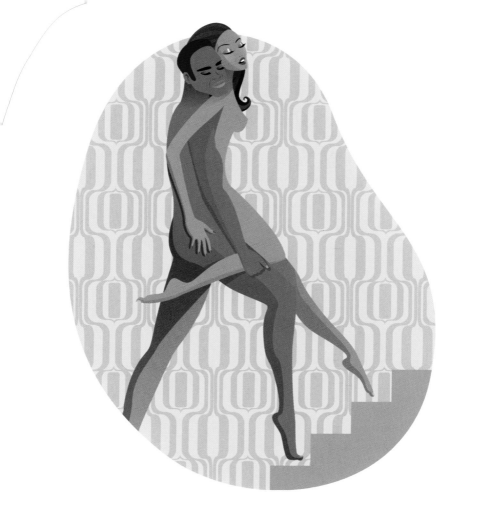

love comes from behind

This is a wonderfully intimate position that can really become part of regular, loving sex. She lies on her front on the bed and raises her buttocks towards him, pushing up slightly onto her knees as he settles himself above her, being careful not to put all his weight on her. She parts her legs and, supporting himself with his elbows or on his hands, he should be able to penetrate her.

It is hard for her to access her clitoris in this position, and maintaining the height of her buttocks, pushing upwards to meet his thrusts, can be tiring. It's a good idea to put pillows or cushions beneath her belly to avoid this. He may be able to reach her clitoris with one hand, reaching in front of one thigh. This is a great position if the man enjoys controlling the depth and pace of the action. She can hardly move, so it is great for a woman who likes to give up control.

Penetration is deep, tight, and may hit her G-spot. The movement his penis is causing may cause her clitoris to rub pleasantly against the pillows or bedding. Nicest of all, this is the one rear-entry position in which it's possible to be really intimate; he can caress her neck and face, kissing her ears, and whispering softly to her.

a rush of blood to the head

This isn't for every day, but it's a novelty, and a bit of fun, that is actually easier than it sounds. She lies on her back on the bed or floor (a firm but somewhat padded surface is best) and puts her hands on her hips. With her elbows beneath her, she pushes up her hips and legs as if she's about to thrust her legs into the air like a gymnast or yogi. He kneels in front of her and, taking hold of her calves or ankles, places her legs on his shoulders so that her ankles are either side of his neck and her feet behind his head.

Penetration can be difficult if he doesn't enjoy angling his erection downwards. Once inside, though, the upper surface of his penis can press pleasurably on her G-spot. It requires you both to be supple.

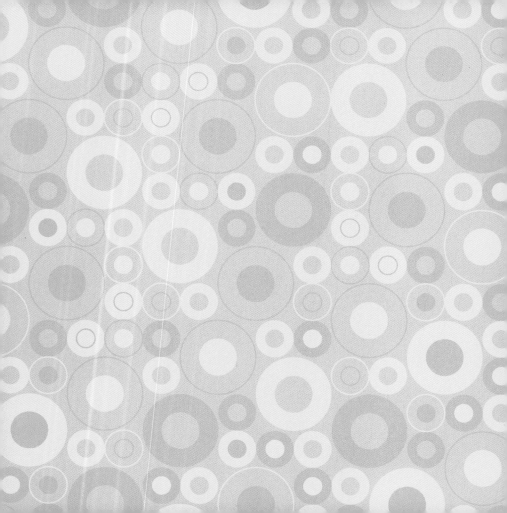

chapter
four

kama sutra
spice

splitting a bamboo

She lies back against a big cushion, and he enters her. She then places one of her legs on her partner's shoulder and stretches the other leg out along the bed. After a few moments she reverses the procedure so the other leg is on his shoulder and her opposite leg stretched out.

turning position

From making love face-to-face, the man turns the woman under him without removing his penis from her vagina, enjoying the feeling of their tangled limbs chafing each other.

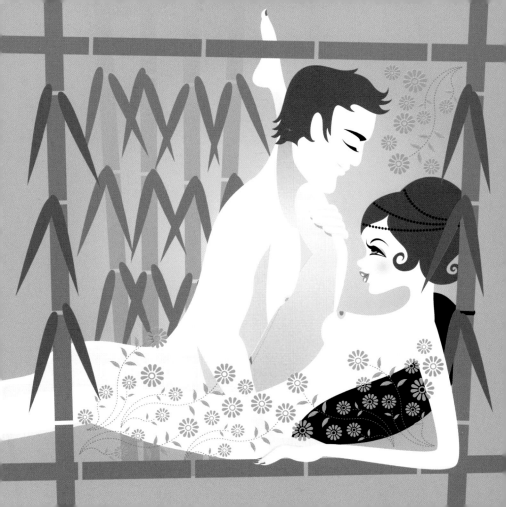

pair of tongs

The woman sits on top of the man with her knees drawn up and her feet placed either side of his hips. She eases herself onto his erect penis and holds it in her by pressing her thighs together. In this position lovemaking can last a long time as deep thrusting is not easily achieved.

self-created position

The man sits with his legs crossed and the woman is on his lap with knees bent and either side of him. She should slightly raise one leg by putting a hand under her foot. By moving her leg around, she can create exquisite sensations.

wheel of kama

The man sits between the legs of the woman, who is lying on her back. He holds her legs wide apart, and he stretches his arms as far as he possibly can on both sides of her. He should move her body around underneath him.

yawning position

She lies back, raises her thighs and keeps them wide apart held at the knee during lovemaking. Good for accommodating a lover with a large penis.

the bow

She lies back with cushions under her hips to raise her sexual parts. Her back should be arched like a bow. Then the man aims his penis into her like an arrow. A very popular position good for all sizes of penis.

opening and blossoming

She lies on her back and lifts both legs straight up, feet pointing to the ceiling. He inserts his penis into her, taking hold of her legs and bringing them together. Their thighs should be pressed very closely together.

the crab

The man and woman both lie on their sides. He lies between her thighs with one of her legs under him and one thrown over him so that she can pull him into her.

packed position

The woman lies down flat, raises her thighs bent at the knee and crosses one leg over the other. He then enters her. This position creates a very snug fit between the penis and vagina, especially if his penis is smaller than her vagina.

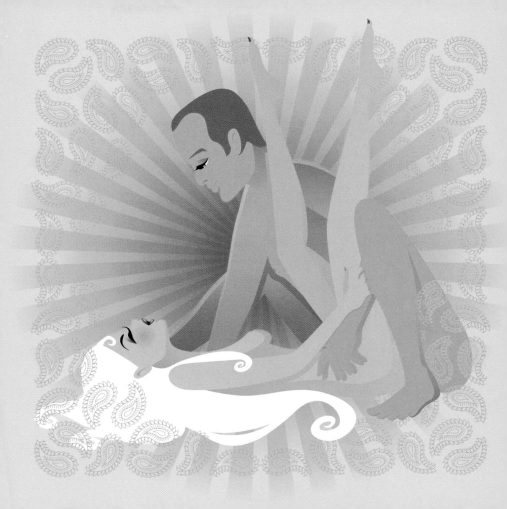

suspended position

The man supports himself against a wall or tree and the woman sits on his joined-together hands with her legs wrapped around his waist, her arms thrown around his neck, and her feet pressing into whatever the man is leaning against. This is ideal for a very strong man and a light woman. For those who find this difficult, a modern interpretation would have the woman sitting on the edge of a table.

the swing

The woman sits on top of the man, who raises his middle so that he can flex himself up and down in a reverse of a push-up. For a variation the woman faces away from him so he has the glorious sight of her buttocks moving up and down.

tantric tortoise

She is underneath him, with her right leg resting on his left shoulder. From this position she should place the soles of both feet into the middle of his chest, imagining herself being created from his heart. He should press her knees with his arms and control his breathing.

elephant position

The woman lies down so her breasts, stomach and thighs are all in contact with the bed. The man then comes from behind to extend himself over her body, caressing her sides and feeling the glorious voluptuousness of her curves. He should enter her with his lower back curved in, working his way into her from underneath.

Meanwhile, she arches her back inwards to propel her vagina into an accessible position. Although she is facing away from him, her movements should be proudly erotic, lewd, and encouraging.

oral techniques

Oral-genital sex requires us to become aware of the natural musky aromas of our partner and relish their individual scent.

penis-loving
Plump up your moistened lips and, with your head at a sideways angle, draw your lips along his penis without actually taking it inside your mouth—a useful alternative for women who gag easily!

vagina-honoring
Like a mouth, it has two lips and a tongue—the clitoris, the starburst pearl of a woman's pleasure. The man should approach the vagina as if he were drinking from a life-giving fountain. This is the place to use the tongue to bring her to a state of climax or arousal.

the infamous "69"
This is the oral position that allows for mutual pleasure. The woman should try to harmonize the movements of her mouth and vagina to the point where her partner loses himself in the all-enveloping essence of the female energies. The close contact of his mouth with her vaginal energy is said to stimulate the pineal and pituitary glands to release chemicals. His erect penis exudes electrical energy that will bring about an exchange of energies that envelop the couple in loving harmony.

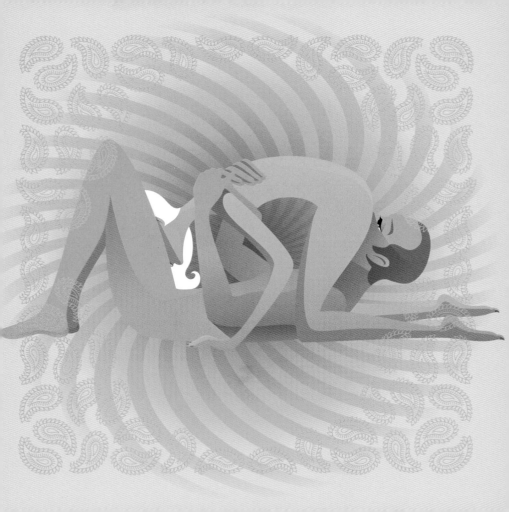

safe sex and loving

Even if you both know you each have a clean bill of sexual health, there's no excuse not to use a condom. The following tips will help you avoid that dreaded moment when the flow of your lovemaking stops as you wrestle with the foil wrapper! Maintain the eroticism between you, and show a bit of style!

A brief genital massage will put him in a mood in which he's likely to maintain an erection. Focusing on his penis as part of your lovemaking will indulge him, turning the condom experience into a treat, not an obligation. Maintain the flow of the massage as you apply the condom. You will tear the latex if you rip the wrapper open with your teeth, so avoid the temptation.

Holding it by the teat at the end to make sure the air is squeezed out, and that it is about to roll in the correct direction down his shaft, rest it on the tip of his penis and roll it down to the base with the other. Don't move straight to placing yourself where he can penetrate you, and don't be hurt if he wants to adjust the condom himself so that his foreskin contracts comfortably, and it remains covering his shaft right to the base.

If condoms are part of your means of avoiding pregnancy and infection, always check the expiry date and use one that conforms to a Federal standard. Novelty condoms aren't designed for contraception or protection.

For a slutty sense of adventure, try putting the condom on with your mouth. A flavored condom will make the experience more pleasant for you, and for him if you're planning on kissing him afterwards! Remove lip-balm, lipstick, or lip-gloss which may contain oils that weaken latex.

Cover your teeth with your lips at all times. Hold the teat of the condom between your pursed lips, sucking inwards lightly to hold it in place. Holding his penis in one closed hand, use your lips to place the condom on its tip. Use your spare hand as necessary to help it down over his glans, and thereafter use your lips and tongue to slide it down the rest of his shaft—a surprisingly deep and sudden feeling for him. Abandon it if and when you can't accommodate any more of him at the back of your throat, and let your hands take over.

index